# Mediterranean Diet for Beginners

Burn fat and reset your metabolism with a meal plan with recipes for weight loss. Gain energy and burn fat for healthy lifestyle.

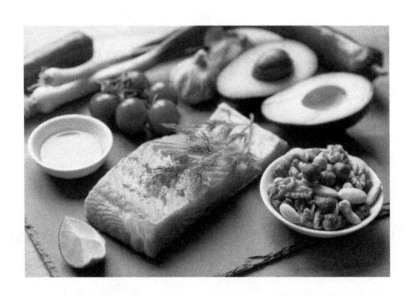

# Table of Contents

# Chapter Four: Breakfast Recipes

Breakfast is one of the most important meals of the day! To set you up for success, I have included several delicious recipes to get you started. Many of these recipes are interchangeable. If you see a fruit that you don't like, feel free to switch it up. One of the best parts of the Mediterranean Diet is flexibility; choose foods that excite you while fueling you at the same time.

# Berry Fruity Yogurt Parfait

Servings: Two

Time: Five Minutes

Calories Per Serving: 290

Carbohydrates: 27g

Proteins: 29g

Fats: 10g

Ingredients:

- Raspberries (1 C.)
- Blackberries (1 C.)
- Plain Greek Yogurt (1.50 C.)
- Walnuts, Chopped (.25 C.)

Instructions:

1. This recipe is incredibly basic. All you will need to do is take your favorite cup or bowl and layer your selected berries with the yogurt. For an added treat, you can sprinkle your favorite nut on top. I enjoy walnuts, but you can choose any for some delicious crunch in your parfait.

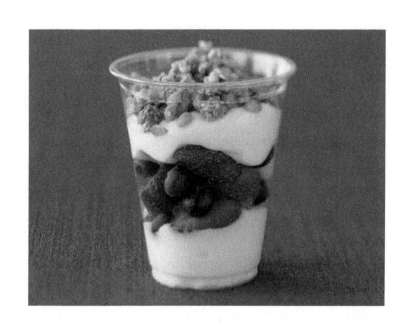

# Banana and Chocolate Vegetarian Smoothie

Servings: Two

Time: Five Minutes

Calories Per Serving: 220

Carbohydrates: 57g

Proteins:2g

Fats: 2g

Ingredients:

- Honey (3 T.)
- Cocoa Powder, unsweetened (3 T.)
- Almond Milk, unsweetened (1 C.)
- Bananas (2)
- Ice (1 C.)

Instructions:

1. For a quick and simple breakfast, toss all of the ingredients from above into a blender. Place your blender on high for about thirty seconds or until smooth.
2. For the leftovers, pop them into the fridge, and you can enjoy it again the next day! If you do this, I recommend placing it in the blender again to assure it is smooth.

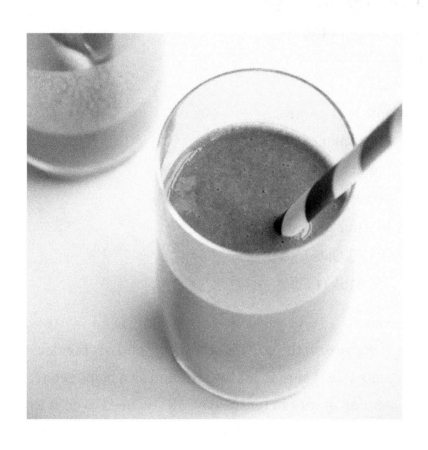

# Strawberry and Oat Breakfast Smoothie

Servings: Two

Time: Five Minutes

Calories Per Serving: 230

Carbohydrates: 45g

Proteins: 8g

Fats: 4g

Ingredients:

- Sweetener of Choice (1.50 t.)
- Vanilla Extract (.50 t.)
- Strawberries, Frozen (15)
- Banana (1)
- Rolled Oats (.50 C.)
- Soy Milk (1 C.)

Instructions:

1. If you are on the go, this strawberry and oat breakfast smoothie is sure to hit the spot and also helps get a serving of fruit in for the day. All you need to do is toss all of the ingredients from above into a blender and blend until smooth. The sugar and vanilla extract are optional but add some sweetness if that is what you are looking for in your breakfast smoothie.

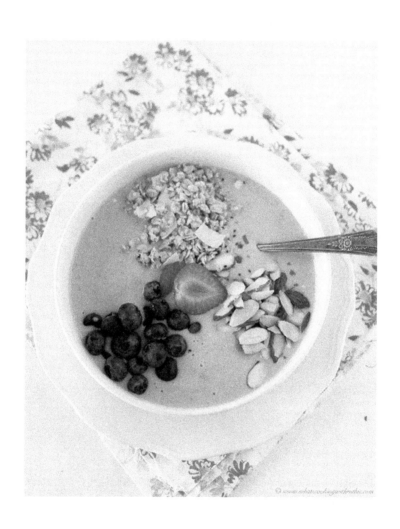

# Breakfast Quinoa

Servings: Four

Time: Twenty-five Minutes

Calories Per Serving: 330

Carbohydrates: 54g

Proteins: 12g

Fats: 8g

Ingredients:

- Dried Apricots (5)
- Dried Dates (2)
- Honey (2 T.)
- Vanilla Extract (1 t.)
- Salt (1 t.)
- Milk (2 C.)
- Quinoa (1 C.)
- Ground Cinnamon (1 t.)
- Almonds (.25 C.)

Instructions:

1. To start off, you will want to place a skillet over medium heat. Once it feels warm, you will want to toast your almonds for just a few minutes. On average, it should take about three to five minutes for them to turn a nice golden color. Once this has happened, you can set them aside

2. Next, you will want to use the same saucepan and add in the quinoa with the one tablespoon of cinnamon. Once it is warm, you can add in the salt and milk. You will want to stir until the mix begins to boil.

3. When it is boiling, reduce the heat to a lower setting and allow the mixture to simmer for fifteen minutes or so. Place a cover over the pan to keep all of the heat in.

4. Once the fifteen minutes are up, you can stir in half of your toasted almonds, the dried apricots, dried dates, vanilla extract, and honey in.

5. When you are ready, place each serving into a bowl and top with the remaining almonds. This dish can be enjoyed warm or cold!

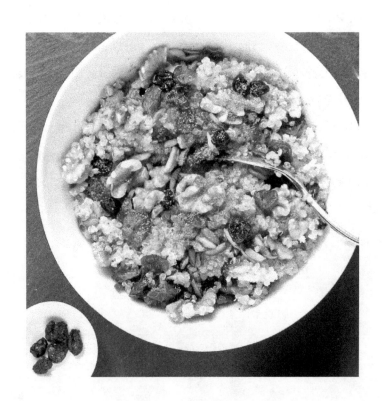

# Healthy Carrot Mini Muffins

Servings: Eighteen

Time: Twenty Minutes

Calories Per Serving: 120 for Two Muffins

Carbohydrates: 20g

Proteins: 2g

Fats: 3g

Ingredients:

- Raisins (.25 C.)
- Carrots, grated (1.50 C.)
- Olive Oil (2 T.)
- Egg (1)
- Honey (2 T.)
- Almond Milk, unsweetened (1.25 C.)
- Salt (.25 t.)
- Nutmeg (.50 t.)
- Ginger (2 t.)
- Cinnamon (2 t.)
- Baking Powder (1 t.)
- Baking Soda (1 t.)
- Brown Sugar (3 T.)
- Old-fashioned Oats (.50 C.)
- All-purpose Flour (.50 C.)
- Whole-wheat Flour (1 C.)

- Oat Bran (1 C.)

Instructions:

1. You will want to start off this recipe by heating your oven to 350 degrees.

2. As the oven heats up, you can prep your muffin tin by coating it with nonstick cooking spray or lining it with paper liners.

3. When this is prepped, take a large bowl and place the flours, oat bran, oats, salt, nutmeg, ginger, cinnamon, baking powder, baking soda, and brown sugar. Once you have done this, you can set it to the side.

4. Next, you will want to take another bowl and mix together the olive oil with the honey, almond milk, and one egg.

5. Once both of these bowls are prepared, you will want to fold the two ingredients together until they are blended. At this point in the recipe, you may notice that the batter will be fairly lumpy with flour streaks still remaining.

6. When this step is completed, you will now want to add in the raisins and carrots.

7. Now that your batter is ready, go ahead and fill the muffin tins up around three-fourths of the way full.

8. With the muffin tins filled, pop it into the oven for fifteen to twenty minutes. Be sure to keep a close eye on the muffins to assure they cook correctly. When they

are cooked through, you should be able to insert a toothpick and retrieve it clean,

9. Once the muffins are done, remove from the oven, allow to cool, and enjoy!

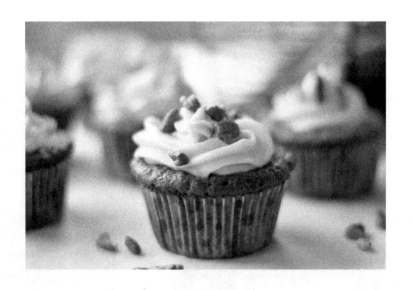

# Spinach Omelet

Servings: One

Time: Fifteen Minutes

Calories Per Serving: 190

Carbohydrates: 3g

Proteins: 17g

Fats: 13g

Ingredients:

- Baby Spinach (1 C.)
- Eggs (2)
- Salt (1 t.)
- Pepper (1 t.)
- Nutmeg (.10 t.)
- Onion Powder (.25 t.)
- Parmesan Cheese, grated (1.50 T.)

Instructions:

1. You can start off by heating a small skillet over medium heat. Use Olive oil to coat the skillet before you begin cooking.
2. While the skillet heats up, you can take a small bowl and begin to beat the eggs until they are mixed together.
3. Once the eggs are mixed, add in the baby spinach and the cheese. If desired, go ahead and season it the way

you would like. I enjoy using nutmeg, onion powder, and basic salt and pepper in mine.

4. When your mixture is complete, add it into the skillet and cook for around three minutes on the one side. When it is cooked through, the edges will look partially set, and you can flip it. I suggest cooking the other side for around two to three minutes or until cooked through.

5. Once cooked through, try reducing the heat to low and cook the omelet for another two to three minutes to achieve a crispy outside and soft inside.

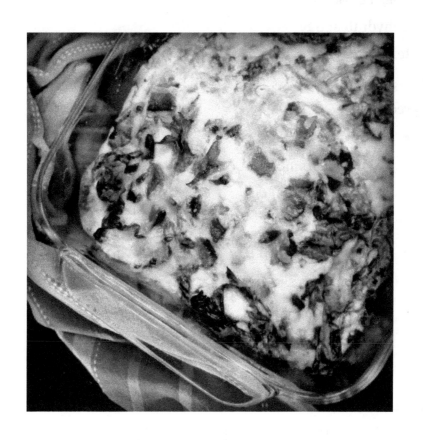

# Veggie Pancakes

Servings: Four

Time: Twenty-five Minutes

Calories Per Serving: 440

Carbohydrates: 82g

Proteins: 21g

Fats: 5g

Ingredients:

- Olive Oil (1 t.)
- Spinach (1 bunch)
- Carrot, shredded (1)
- Salt (1 t.)
- Palm Sugar (1.50 T)
- Ginger Root, sliced (1)
- Water (3 C.)
- Dry Yellow Lentils (1.25 C.)
- Rice (1 C.)

Instructions:

1. To prepare for this recipe, I suggest you get the rice and lentils prepared the day before. You will want to soak these for four to five hours.

2. Once this is done, you will want to place the lentils and rice into a food processor with the salt, palm sugar, and ginger. When this mixture is smooth, you can toss in

the spinach and carrot as well. I suggest blending until you are satisfied with the smoothness.

3. When you have your mixture, you can go ahead and place a skillet over medium heat. Once warm, spread the batter onto the skillet and cook like a regular pancake.

4. On average, these vegetable pancakes will take around fifteen minutes. You will be able to tell they are ready to flip when you see the edges begin to set. When you see this, go ahead and cook the other side until it has turned brown.

5. Remove the pancakes from the skillet and enjoy for a healthy breakfast!

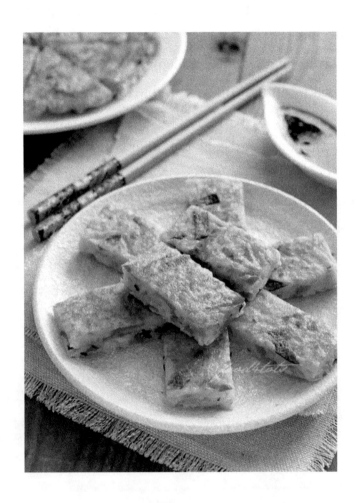

# Zucchini Breakfast Pizza

Servings: One

Time: Forty Minutes

Calories Per Serving: 270

Carbohydrates: 36g

Proteins: 12g

Fats: 11g

Ingredients:

- Maple Syrup (1 t.)
- Orange Zest (.25 t.)
- Banana (.50)
- Grapes (4)
- Strawberries (2)
- Greek Yogurt (.25 C.)
- Vanilla Extract (.10 t.)
- Maple Syrup (1.50 t.)
- Egg (1)
- Zucchini, shredded (.50 C.)
- Cinnamon (.10 t.)
- Coconut Flour (2 T.)

Instructions:

1. You will want to begin this recipe by heating your oven to 350 degrees. While this warms up, you can get a baking sheet all set by lining it with parchment paper.

2. Now that your tools are set up, take a small bowl and mix the cinnamon with the coconut flour. Once this is done, you will want to add in the vanilla extract, one and a half teaspoons of real maple syrup, the one egg, and your shredded zucchini.

3. Be sure to mix everything together well. When you are satisfied with the consistency, place the mixture onto your prepared baking sheet and form what you think resembles a pizza crust.

4. When you are ready, pop the baking sheet into the oven with your crust. Leave this in there for around fifteen minutes or until it looks like it is cooked through. When it looks good to you, remove the crust from the oven and allow to cool completely.

5. Once the crust is cooled, go ahead and spread the yogurt over the top like you would with sauce for a pizza.

6. Now, it is time to go crazy with the fruits! I enjoy using banana, grapes, and strawberries but you can really use any fruit you would like.

7. For some extra flavor, use some orange zest and drizzle maple syrup over the whole thing. This "pizza" is an

excellent way to add a serving of fruit and vegetable to your day!

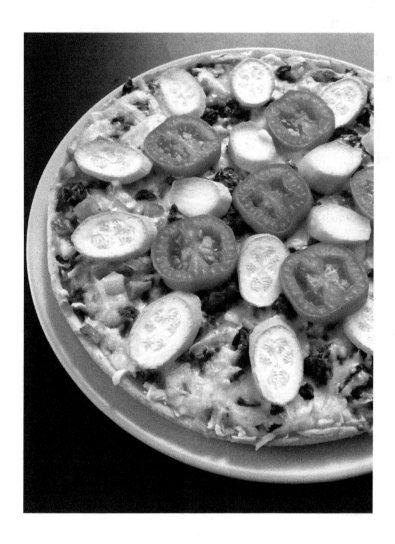

# Black Bean Bowl Breakfast

Servings: Two

Time: Fifteen Minutes

Calories Per Serving: 630

Carbohydrates: 47g

Proteins: 28g

Fats: 39g

Ingredients:

- Salsa (.25 C.)
- Avocado (1)
- Black Beans (1 Can)
- Eggs (4)
- Olive Oil (2 T.)
- Salt (1 t.)
- Pepper (1 t.)

Instructions:

1. To begin, you will want to heat a small pan over medium heat. As this warms up, pour in your two tablespoons of olive oil and allow it to warm up.
2. Once the olive oil is warm, go ahead and stir in your eggs and allow them to cook. This process should take about three to five minutes to cook through.
3. When the eggs are cooked through, you will want to remove them from the heat and turn the oven off.

4. Now, place your black beans into a microwave-safe bowl and cook them until the beans are warm. Typically, this should only take about a minute.
5. When you are ready, divide the beans into two bowls and place the scrambled eggs on top.
6. For extra flavor, top the bowls off with avocado and salsa. Finally, season with salt and pepper to taste and you have a delicious and healthy breakfast in your hands.

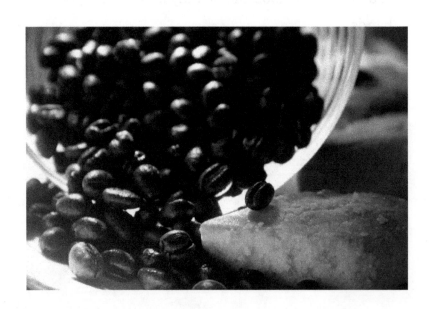

# Breakfast Zucchini Pie

Servings: Eight

Time: One Hour

Calories Per Serving: 240

Carbohydrates: 14g

Proteins: 7g

Fats: 18g

Ingredients:

- Parsley, chopped (1 t.)
- Dried Marjoram (.50 t.)
- Parmesan Cheese (.50 C.)
- Olive Oil (.50 C.)
- Whole Wheat Baking Mix (1 C.)
- Eggs (4)
- Onion (1)
- Zucchini (3 C.)
- Salt (1 t.)
- Pepper (1 t.)

Instructions:

1. You can begin this recipe by heating your oven to 350 degrees. While this warms up, you will want to grease a baking pan or a pie plate with some olive oil.
2. When your tools are ready, take a mixing bowl and combine the marjoram, parmesan cheese, olive oil,

baking mix, eggs, onion, zucchini, and pepper together. Be sure to mix everything together well before pouring into your baking dish.

3. Once ready, pop the dish into the oven for about thirty minutes. When it is cooked through, the top should be lightly browned.

4. Remove from the oven when it is done and allow to cool. Slice it up into servings and enjoy a warm breakfast.

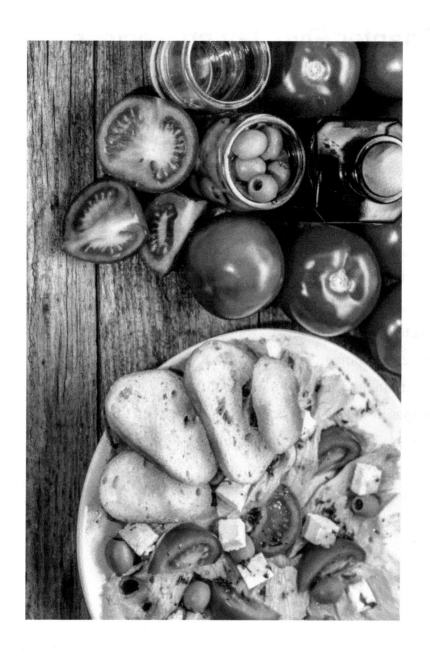

# Chapter Five: Lunch Recipes

Are you feeling hungry yet? As you can see, being on a diet doesn't always mean that your meals are going to be bland! Whether you are enjoying a delicious breakfast parfait or baking a zucchini pie for your family; there is a recipe for just about anyone! As you can tell, you can always get a serving of fruit or vegetable into just about any meal!

Now, we will dive into some simple lunch recipes for you to try. In these meals, we will begin to introduce some lean proteins. Remember that you want to keep these to a minimum as you start to plan out your meals. Many of these recipes are filled with vegetables, try to keep that your main focus. When you feel confident enough with your cooking talents, you can always start adding your own twists to the recipes to follow. It's all about flexibility!

# Harvest Salad

Servings: Six

Time: Fifteen Minutes

Calories Per Serving: 340

Carbohydrates: 22g

Proteins: 7g

Fats: 27g

Ingredients:

- Walnut Oil (.33 C.)
- Red Wine Vinegar (2 T.)
- Red Raspberry Jam (2 T.)
- Red Onion (.50)
- Avocado (1)
- Blue Cheese (.50 C.)
- Dried Cranberries (.50 C.)
- Spinach (1 Bunch)
- Walnuts (.50 C.)
- Salt (1 t.)
- Pepper (1 t.)

Instructions:

1. Before you begin assembling your salad, you will want to preheat your oven to 375 degrees. When it is ready, you can toast your walnuts in the oven for five minutes.

2. While the walnuts cook, begin to toss the other ingredients together. Add in the red onion, avocado, tomatoes (if desired), blue cheese, cranberries, and spinach. Remember that the Mediterranean diet is all about vegetables; the more, the merrier!

3. Once your walnuts are done, remove them from the oven and allow to cool for a few minutes. Once cooled, you can toss them into your salad.

4. To make the dressing, take another small bowl and mix together the walnut oil, red wine vinegar, and raspberry jam. For extra flavor, feel free to flavor your home-made dressing with salt and pepper.

5. Finally, pour the dressing over the salad and give the salad a good toss before serving.

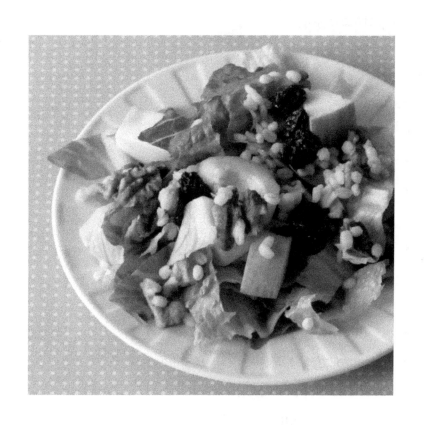

# Vegetarian Chili

Servings: Eight

Time: One Hour

Calories Per Serving: 150

Carbohydrates: 30g

Proteins: 7g

Fats: 3g

Ingredients:

- Dried Basil (1.50 t.)
- Dried Oregano (1.50 t.)
- Cumin (1 T.)
- Whole Kernel Corn (1 Can)
- Kidney Beans (1 Can)
- Peeled Tomatoes (1 Can)
- Mushrooms (1.50 C.)
- Chili Powder (1 T.)
- Celery (.75 C.)
- Red Bell Pepper (1 C.)
- Green Bell Pepper (1 C.)
- Carrots (.75 C.)
- Onion (1 C.)
- Olive Oil (1 T.)

Instructions:

1. To begin this recipe, you will want to take a large saucepan and place it over medium heat. As it begins to warm up, you will want to place your olive oil and allow it to sizzle.

2. When the olive oil is warm, place the garlic, carrots, and onions and allow to cook until they are tender. Once those are set you can add in the celery, red pepper, green pepper, and spice it all up with the chili powder. This will probably take around six minutes to get the vegetables nice and tender for your chili.

3. Next, stir in the mushrooms, kidney beans, corn, and tomatoes. You can cook these for four or five minutes.

4. Finally, season all of the vegetables with basil, oregano, and cumin. Once this is done, you can go ahead and bring this mixture to a boil.

5. When the pan begins to boil, reduce the heat to medium and place a cover over the top. Allow the mixture to simmer for twenty minutes or so. Be sure to stir the pan occasionally, so nothing burns to the bottom.

6. Finally, remove from the heat and enjoy your healthy lunch.

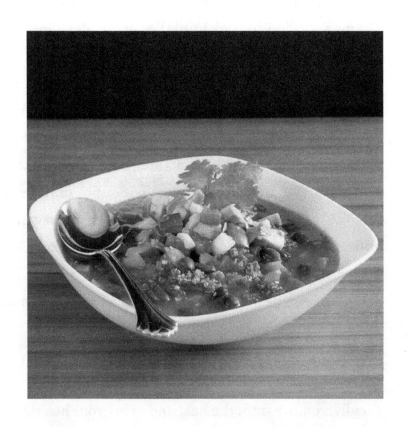

# Lentil Soup

Servings: Four

Time: One and a Half Hours

Calories Per Serving: 360

Carbohydrates: 40g

Proteins: 16g

Fats: 16g

Ingredients:

- Red Wine Vinegar (1 t.)
- Olive Oil (1 t.)
- Salt (1 t.)
- Pepper (1 t.)
- Tomato Paste (1 T.)
- Bay Leaves (2)
- Dried Rosemary (1 t.)
- Oregano (1 t.)
- Water (1 Q.)
- Carrot (1)
- Onion (1)
- Minced Garlic (1 T.)
- Olive Oil (.25 C.)
- Brown Lentils (8 oz.)

Instructions:

1. To start, you will want to place a large saucepan over high heat. Once in place, you can pour in the lentils and cover with water. Bring the saucepan to a boil and cook the lentils for around ten minutes. After this time, drain and place to the side.

2. Next, you will want to place a saucepan over medium heat. Once it begins to warm up, add in your olive oil and allow that to heat up. When the olive oil begins to sizzle, toss in your carrot, onion, and garlic and cook for about five minutes. By the end, the onion should be translucent.

3. Next, you will want to pour in the cook lentils, bay leaves, rosemary, oregano, and the quart of water. Bring everything to a boil and then reduce the heat to medium-low. You will want this mixture to simmer for around ten minutes or so.

4. After ten minutes have passed, you will want to stir in the tomato paste and season with the salt and pepper to taste. Once this step is complete, you will want to place the cover back on and allow it to cook for thirty to forty minutes. Be sure to stir the pot and add additional water if needed.

5. Finally, drizzle in olive oil and red wine vinegar for extra flavor before serving for lunch or dinner.

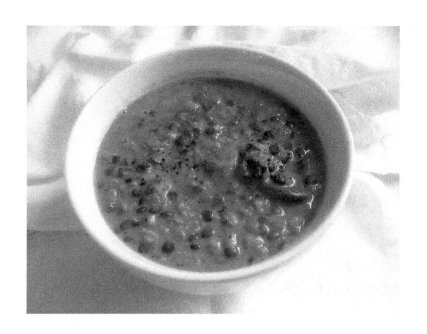

# Greek Quinoa Salad

Servings: Ten

Time: Two Hours

Calories Per Serving: 227

Carbohydrates: 26g

Proteins: 8g

Fats: 11g

Ingredients:

- Lemon (1)
- Salt (1 t.)
- Pepper (1 t.)
- Garlic (2)
- Red Wine Vinegar (3 T.)
- Olive Oil (3 T.)
- Feta Cheese (4 oz.)
- Red Onion (.50 C.)
- Parsley (.75 C.)
- Olives (.50 C.)
- Grape Tomatoes (1 C.)
- Quinoa (2 C.)
- Chicken Broth (3.50 C.)

Instructions:

1.  To start, bring a saucepan over high heat. Once placed, pour in the broth and quinoa and allow the mixture to come to a boil. When it begins to boil, you will want to lower the heat to medium-low, cover the pot, and allow the quinoa to simmer for fifteen to twenty minutes. By the end, the quinoa should absorb all of the water. Once this has happened, remove the saucepan from the oven and set aside in a large bowl.

2.  As the quinoa cools down, you will want to add in the garlic, vinegar, olive oil, feta cheese, onion, olives, parsley, and tomato in.

3.  If desired, try to squeeze some lemon juice over the salad for extra flavoring. You can also season with salt and pepper. I also suggest you chill the salad in the fridge for at least an hour before you enjoy. This makes an excellent side salad with your choice of lean protein or vegetable.

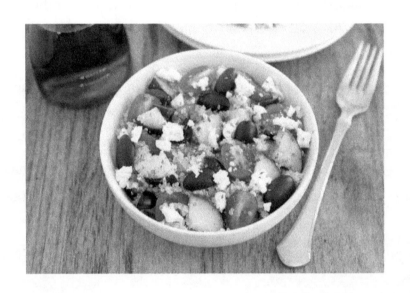

# Mediterranean Lemon Chicken

Servings: Four

Time: One and a Half Hours

Calories Per Serving: 520

Carbohydrates: 65g

Proteins: 30g

Fats: 17g

Ingredients:

- Lemon (1)
- Red Onion (1)
- Red Bell Pepper (1)
- Red Potatoes (8)
- Chicken Breast, boneless and skinless (4)
- Pepper (.50 t.)
- Salt (1 t.)
- Oregano (1 T.)
- Garlic Cloves (4)
- Lemon Zest (2 T.)
- Lemon Juice (2 T.)
- Olive Oil (.25 C.)

Instructions:

1. Begin this recipe by heating your oven to 400 degrees.

2. As the oven heats up, you will want to take a small bowl so that you can combine the black pepper, salt, oregano, garlic, lemon zest, lemon juice, and your olive oil.

3. Once these are well combined, brush the lemon juice over your chicken. You will want to place the chicken on a baking dish.

4. Next, you will want to prepare your lemon, red onion, red bell pepper, and potatoes by slicing them into bite-sized pieces. Once this is done, you can place them in the bowl and pour the remaining lemon mixture over top of them. You will want to make sure you toss the vegetables, so they are evenly coated by the lemon juice.

5. When this is done, you will want to arrange your vegetables around the chicken on the baking dish.

6. Once everything is in place, pop the dish into the oven for thirty minutes or so. You will want to cook until the chicken is browned, and vegetables appear tender.

7. Remove the dish from the oven, allow to cool, and enjoy!

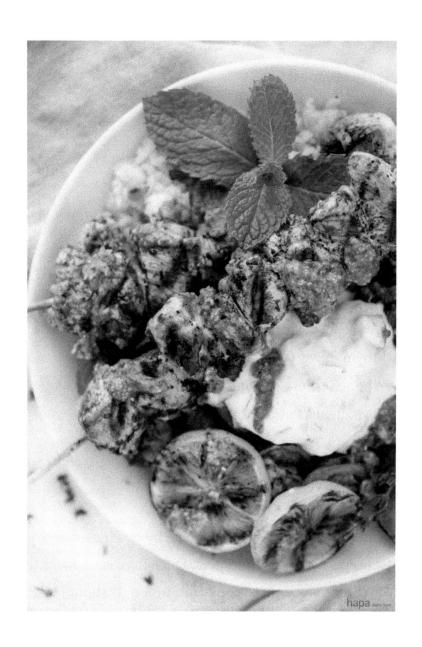

# Corn and Black Bean Quesadilla

Servings: Eight

Time: Forty Minutes

Calories Per Serving: 365

Carbohydrates: 46g

Proteins: 14g

Fats: 15g

Ingredients:

- Whole Wheat Tortillas (8)
- Monterey Jack Cheese (1.50 C.)
- Butter (2 T.)
- Salsa (.25 C.)
- Brown Sugar (1 T.)
- Whole Kernel Corn (1 Can)
- Black Beans (1 Can)
- Onion (3 T.)
- Olive Oil (2 t.)

Instructions:

1. You will want to start this recipe by placing a large saucepan over medium heat. Once in place, toss in the olive oil and begin to cook your onion. It should take about two minutes for the onion to become tender.
2. When the onion is cooked through, add in the sugar, pepper, salsa, corn, and the black beans. You will want

to cook this mixture for around three minutes or until cooked through. Once this is done, remove the mixture from the heat and place to the side.

3. In a large skillet, melt the butter over medium heat. When this is done, place your whole wheat tortilla in and sprinkle cheese on top. Once in place, add in the bean mixture and then place another tortilla on top.

4. Once the quesadilla is assembled, you will want to cook each side until they turn a nice golden color. Feel free to add more butter as needed.

5. When both sides are golden, slice into pieces, and your meal is ready.

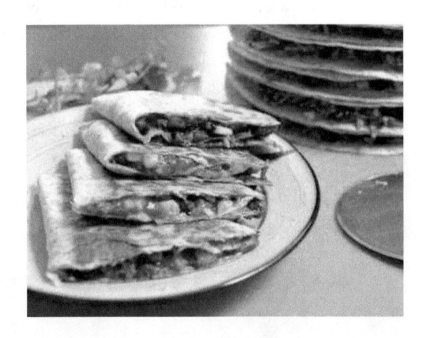

# Cucumber Sandwich

Servings: One

Time: Ten Minutes

Calories Per Serving: 500

Carbohydrates: 47g

Proteins: 12g

Fats: 33g

Ingredients:

- Avocado (.50)
- Pepperoncini (1 oz.)
- Lettuce (1)
- Tomato (1)
- Red Wine Vinegar (1 t.)
- Olive Oil (1 t.)
- Alfalfa Sprouts (2 T.)
- Cucumber (6 Slices)
- Cream Cheese (2 T.)
- Whole Wheat Bread (2 Slices)

Instructions:

1. First, you will want to spread one tablespoon of cream cheese on each slice of bread.
2. Once this is complete, you will want to arrange the cucumber and sprouts on top of one another.

3. For extra flavor, try to sprinkle the olive oil and red wine vinegar over the cucumber.
4. Next, layer the lettuce, tomato, and pepperoncini on top.
5. Finally, spread the avocado on the other slice of bread, and your sandwich is ready to be served.

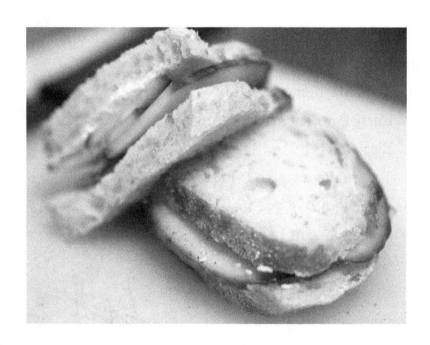

# Sweet and Spicy Chicken Salad Sandwich

Servings: Eight

Time: Forty-five

Calories Per Serving: 230

Carbohydrates: 13g

Proteins: 15g

Fats: 14g

Ingredients:

- Light Mayonnaise (.75 C.)
- Curry Powder (.50 t.)
- Black Pepper (.50 t.)
- Toasted Pecans (.50 C.)
- Green Grapes (.33 C.)
- Golden Raisins (.33 C.)
- Golden Delicious Apple (1)
- Green Onions (4)
- Celery (1)
- Chicken Breast, boneless and skinless (4)

Instructions:

1. Start off by preparing all of the ingredients from above. Be sure that they are clean and chopped into small, bite-sized pieces.

2. Once ready, you can take a large bowl and combine all of the ingredients from above. You can vary the pepper and curry powder according to your own taste,

3. When everything is combined, serve on your favorite bread and lunch is ready.

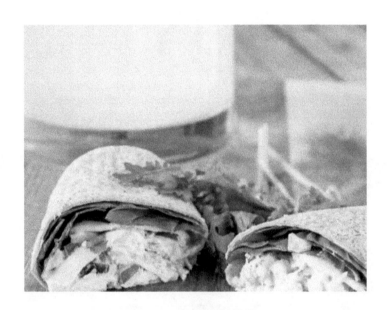

# Egg and Shrimp Salad

Servings: Four

Time: Fifteen Minutes

Calories Per Serving: 290

Carbohydrates: 2g

Proteins: 31g

Fats: 18g

Ingredients:

- Lettuce (4)
- Fresh Dill (1)
- Dijon Mustard (1 t.)
- Mayonnaise (4 T.)
- Eggs (4)
- Cooked Shrimp (1 lb.)

Instructions:

1. Before you assemble the salad, you will want to hard-boil your eggs and cook your shrimp. You will want to do this according to their packages.
2. Once cooked, take a large bowl and combine the mayonnaise, Dijon mustard, hard-boiled eggs, and cooked shrimp.
3. You can serve this on your favorite bread, in a pita pocket, or enjoy it on top of a salad!

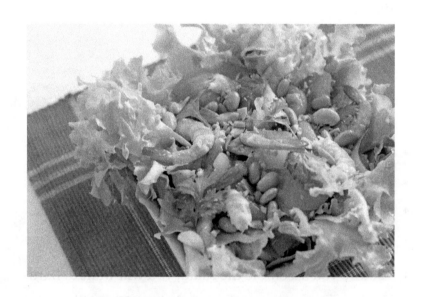

# Dijon Salmon

Servings: Four

Time: Forty Minutes

Calories Per Serving: 420

Carbohydrates: 18g

Proteins: 25g

Fats: 30g

Ingredients:

- Lemon (1)
- Salt (1 t.)
- Pepper (1 t.)
- Salmon Fillet (4)
- Parsley (4 t.)
- Pecans (.25 C.)
- Bread Crumbs (.25 C.)
- Honey (1.50 T.)
- Dijon Mustard (3 T.)
- Butter (.25 C.)

Instructions:

1. Start this recipe off by heating your oven to 400 degrees.
2. As the oven heats up, go ahead and take a small bowl so you can combine the honey, mustard, and butter together.

3. In a separate bowl, you will want to combine the parsley, pecans, and bread crumbs.

4. When you are ready, lay the salmon fillets on a greased baking sheet and brush each fillet with the honey mixture. Once this is done, you can sprinkle the bread crumb mixture over the top of each fillet.

5. Once the oven is heated, place the salmon in for twelve to fifteen minutes. When it is cooked through, the fish will flake easily under a fork.

6. For added flavor, add some salt and pepper. You can also use lemon as a garnish. Serve hot with your favorite vegetable on the side or top of a salad for a well-rounded meal.

# Chapter Six: Dinner Recipes

Next, we move onto some delicious dinner recipes. As you could probably tell, the lunch recipes were fairly light. They are excellent to try if you are short on time and are looking to eat healthily. If weight loss is a goal of yours, I suggest trying meal prep, so these delicious meals are ready to go without much effort when you are short on time.

The dinner recipes to follow will require a bit more time and effort. It should be noted that with more effort will come more flavor. From salmon dishes to chicken dishes, these recipes are filled with delicious flavors and nutrients for you and your family.

# Italian White Bean Soup

Servings: Four

Time: One Hour

Calories Per Serving: 250

Carbohydrates: 38g

Proteins: 12g

Fats: 5g

Ingredients:

- Lemon Juice (1 T.)
- Spinach (1 Bunch)
- Water (2 C.)
- Dried Thyme (.10 t.)
- Black Pepper (.10 t.)
- Chicken Broth (1 Can)
- White Kidney Cans (2 Cans)
- Garlic (1)
- Celery (1)
- Onion (1)
- Olive Oil (1 T.)

Instructions:

1. To begin this recipe, take a large saucepan and begin to heat the olive oil. Once the olive oil starts to sizzle, you will want to add in the celery and onion and cook these

for five to eight minutes. By the end, the vegetables should be tender.

2. Once tender, add in the garlic and continue to cook the mixture for thirty seconds or so. After this time, add in the pepper, thyme, cups of water, beans, and the chicken broth.

3. When everything is in place, bring the mixture to a boil before you reduce the heat and allow everything to simmer for around fifteen minutes.

4. After fifteen minutes, you will want to use a slotted spoon to remove the beans and vegetables from the soup.

5. Next, take a blender and blend the remaining soup until it is smooth. Once the soup mixture is smooth, you can pour it back into the stock and stir in any leftover beans.

6. Finally, bring the pot back to a boil and stir in your spinach. After a minute, the spinach will begin to wilt, and you can add in your lemon juice.

7. For a final touch, try adding fresh Parmesan cheese on top, and your soup is ready to be served.

# Mediterranean Stew for Slow Cooker

Servings: Ten

Time: Ten Hours

Calories Per Serving: 122

Carbohydrates: 31g

Proteins: 4g

Fats: 1g

Ingredients:

- Paprika (.25 t.)
- Ground Cinnamon (.25 t.)
- Crushed Red Pepper (.25 t.)
- Ground Turmeric (.50 t.)
- Ground Cumin (.50 t.)
- Garlic (1)
- Raisins (.50 C.)
- Vegetable Broth (.50 C.)
- Carrot (1)
- Tomato (1)
- Onion (1 C.)
- Frozen Okra (1 Package)
- Tomato Sauce (1 Can)
- Zucchini (2 C.)
- Eggplant (2 C.)
- Butternut Squash (1)

Instructions:

1. You will want to start off this recipe by preparing all of the vegetables from the list above. Be sure to clean them well, peel, and then dice into bite-sized pieces.

2. Once this is complete, place everything into your slow cooker. If desired, season with the paprika, cinnamon, red pepper, turmeric, and cumin to taste.

3. Finally, pop a cover over your slow cooker and cook on a low temperature from eight to ten hours for max flavor. If you are looking to cook it sooner, try placing the slow cooker on high for four to six hours. By the end, the vegetables should be tender and delicious.

# Spaghetti Squash Boats

Servings: Four

Time: Two Hours

Calories Per Serving: 423

Carbohydrates: 22g

Proteins: 18g

Fats: 31g

Ingredients:

- Fresh Parsley (1 T.)
- Tomato (1)
- Salt (.25 t.)
- Lemon Pepper (.25 t.)
- Feta Cheese (4 oz.)
- Italian Seasoning (1 T.)
- Red Bell Pepper (1)
- Zucchini (1)
- Garlic (3)
- Spring Onions (2)
- Italian Sausage Links (3) (Optional)
- Olive Oil (2 T.)
- Spaghetti Squash (1)

Instructions:

1. To start off, you will want to preheat your oven to 350 degrees. While this warms up, you will want to prepare a large baking dish by coating it in tin foil or spraying it down with cooking spray.

2. Once this is done, you will want to prepare your red bell pepper, zucchini, onion, and tomato by dicing them into small, bite-sized pieces. With those all set, you will also be cutting your spaghetti squash down the center to prepare them for the dish.

3. When the oven is ready, you will set the spaghetti squash by itself in the baking dish and pop it in the oven for forty-five minutes. When this time is up, the squash should be tender enough to pierce with a fork. At this point, you will want to turn the squash over and cook it on the other side for five minutes or so.

4. When the squash is ready, you can remove it from the oven. When it cools down a bit, scrape the insides from the skin of the squash and place the insides in a large bowl.

5. Once this is done, you will want to cook the Italian sausage. As you know, red meat should be limited while following the Mediterranean Diet. If you have already hit your max for the week, feel free to substitute the red meat with leaner meat or leave it out altogether!

6. Next, you will take a medium-size skillet and place it over medium heat. Once you have added a tablespoon

of olive oil, you can add in the onion and garlic. Stir these around for five minutes or until the onions are soft. This usually takes around five minutes or so. Once the onions are done, add in the red bell pepper, zucchini, and Italian seasoning. Be sure you continue to stir, so nothing burns to the bottom. These vegetables should be done in around five minutes or so.

7. When your vegetables are done, you will want to stir in the spaghetti squash and feta cheese. You will continue to stir until the cheese has melted. If you have the sausage, you can stir that in last.

8. Finally, season the whole mix with lemon pepper and salt. If desired, add tomato and parsley on top of the boats for some extra flavor. Pour everything back into the skin of the squash and your meal is ready to be served.

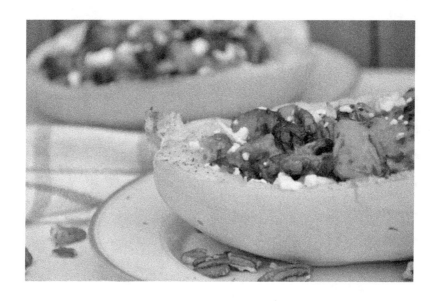

# Baked Zucchini and Potatoes

Servings: Four

Time: Two Hours

Calories Per Serving: 525

Carbohydrates: 66g

Proteins: 12g

Fats: 29g

Ingredients:

- Olive Oil (.50 C.)
- Salt (.25 t.)
- Pepper (.25 t.)
- Fresh Parsley (2 T.)
- Tomatoes (6)
- Red Onions (4)
- Zucchini (4)
- Potatoes (2 Lbs.)

Instructions:

1. Before you begin prepping this recipe, you will want to preheat your oven to 400 degrees.

2. While the oven warms up, you will want to prepare the vegetables for this recipe. First, peel the potatoes and slice them into thin slices. You will want to do the same for the zucchini and red onions.

3. When this step is done, take a large baking dish and spread out the vegetables from above in layers. Once in place, you can cover them with the tomatoes, parsley, and your olive oil. If desired, flavor the dish with salt and pepper to taste. Feel free to toss everything together to assure the vegetables are evenly coated.

4. When you are ready, place the dish into the oven. After an hour, you will want to stir the vegetables to check on them. In the end, the vegetables should be tender, and all of the moisture within the dish will evaporate. Usually, this dish takes around ninety minutes.

5. Once the dish is done, remove from the oven and allow to cool before serving.

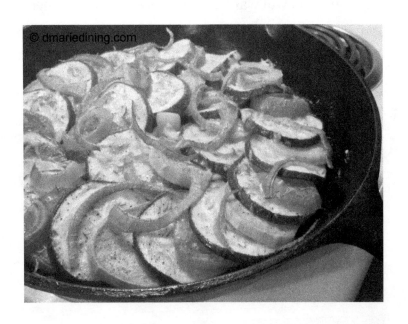

# Baked Spinach and Feta Pita

Servings: Six

Time: Twenty Minutes

Calories Per Serving: 350

Carbohydrates: 42g

Proteins: 12g

Fats: 17g

Ingredients:

- Olive Oil (3 T.)
- Black Pepper (.25 t.)
- Grated Parmesan Cheese (2 T.)
- Feta Cheese (.50 C.)
- Mushrooms (4)
- Spinach (1 Bunch)
- Plum Tomatoes (2)
- Whole Wheat Pita Bread (6)
- Sun-dried Tomato Pesto (1)

Instructions:

1. Before you begin prepping this recipe, you will want to preheat your oven to 350 degrees.
2. As the oven begins to warm up, set up the pita bread and spread a thin layer of pesto on one side of each slice of bread.

3. When this is done, you can set the pita on a baking sheet and layer the pita with the spinach, mushrooms, and tomatoes. Once in place, drizzle on your olive oil and layer the parmesan cheese and feta on cheese. For some extra flavor, feel free to flavor with pepper or any of your favorite spices.

4. Once fully prepared, place the baking sheet in the oven for about twelve minutes. At the end, the pita bread should be crisp and melted.

5. Finally, pull the baking sheet out of the oven and allow the pita bread to cool. You can cut the pitas into quarters for sharing purposes or enjoy them whole!

# Greek Chicken with Pasta

Servings: Six

Time: Thirty Minutes

Calories Per Serving:

Carbohydrates: 70g

Proteins: 33g

Fats: 12g

Ingredients:

- Lemons (2)
- Salt (.25 t.)
- Pepper (.25 t)
- Dried Oregano (2 t.)
- Lemon Juice (2 T.)
- Fresh Parsley (3 T.)
- Feta Cheese (.50 C.)
- Tomato (1)
- Artichoke Hearts (1 Can)
- Chicken Breast, boneless and skinless (1 Lb.)
- Garlic (2)
- Olive Oil (1 T.)
- Red Onion (.50 C.)
- Linguine Pasta (1 Package)

Instructions:

1. To begin, you will want to cook your pasta. I enjoy using linguine for this recipe, but you can use whatever pasta you like best. You will want to try to find whole wheat pasta to enjoy the added health benefits. Once you have your pasta, cook it in a boiling pot of water for eight to ten minutes, or until it is cooked through. When it is done, drain out the water and place the pasta to the side.

2. Next, you will want to begin to heat a large skillet over a medium to high heat. As the pan warms up, add in the olive oil and wait until it begins to sizzle. Once it is warm, add in the onion and garlic. You will want to cook these for two minutes or until it becomes fragrant.

3. Once the onions are tender, add in the chicken and cook until it is no longer pink. You can tell the chicken is cooked when the juices begin to run clear. Typically, this process will take six or seven minutes.

4. When your chicken is cooked, you will want to reduce the heat to a medium-low. Once this is done, you can add in the cooked pasta, artichoke hearts, lemon juice, parsley, oregano, tomato, and the feta cheese.

5. Be sure to continue stirring as you cook your meal. You will want to stir for another three or four minutes to assure everything is cooked through.

6. Finally, remove the pan from the heat and season with salt and pepper if you desire. I also enjoy using the

sliced lemon wedge as a garnish for some extra flair. Allow the meat to cool slightly and then it will be ready to be served.

# Greek Chicken Shish Kebabs

Servings: Six

Time: Two Hours and Thirty Minutes

Calories Per Serving: 290

Carbohydrates: 10g

Proteins: 34g

Fats: 13g

Ingredients:

- Mushrooms (12)
- Cherry Tomatoes (12)
- Onion (1)
- Green Bell Pepper (1)
- Red Bell Pepper (1)
- Wooden Skewers (6)
- Chicken Breast, boneless and skinless (2 Lbs.)
- Black Pepper (.25 t.)
- Salt (.25 t.)
- Dried Thyme (.50 t.)
- Dried Oregano (1 t.)
- Garlic (2)
- White Vinegar (.25 C.)
- Lemon Juice (.25 C.)
- Olive Oil (.25 C.)

Instructions:

1. Before you begin this recipe, you will need to set aside about two hours to properly make the chicken marinate. You will do this by taking a small bowl and mixing together the vinegar, lemon juice, and olive oil with the black pepper, salt, thyme, oregano, and cumin. When these are mixed together, you can add in the chicken and toss it a few times to evenly coat it. I suggest covering it with plastic wrap and placing into the fridge for at least two hours. This gives the juices plenty of time to soak into the chicken.

2. While the marinate is soaking, you will also want to soak the wooden skewers for the kabobs in water. I suggest doing this at least thirty minutes before you use them.

3. When you are ready, take a medium skillet of medium to high heat and place olive oil in. As the olive oil heats up, you can begin to thread the chicken onto the wooden skewers along with the bell pepper slices, onion, mushrooms, and cherry tomatoes. Of course, these are only suggestions. If you have other vegetables like zucchini or squash that you enjoy more, you can substitute just about any vegetable! It is all about what you enjoy most.

4. Once the skewers are ready, you can place them in the skillet and allow them to cook. You will want to make

sure you turn them frequently so that they can brown on all sides. Be sure that the chicken is cooked through and no longer pink in the center. Usually, this takes ten to fifteen minutes.

5. After everything is cooked through, remove the skewers from the heat and allow to cool. This is a fun way to get a serving of protein and vegetable into your day. You can eat them alone or serve with a side of rice.

# Shrimp and Penne

Servings: Eight

Time: Forty Minutes

Calories Per Serving: 385

Carbohydrates: 49g

Proteins: 25g

Fats: 9g

Ingredients:

- Grated Parmesan Cheese (1 C.)
- Shrimp (1 Lb.)
- Diced Tomatoes (2 Cans)
- White Wine (.25 C.)
- Garlic (1 T.)
- Red Onion (.25 C.)
- Olive Oil (2 T.)
- Penne Pasta (1 Package)

Instructions:

1. You can begin by cooking your pasta. For this recipe, I enjoy using penne, but you can use whichever you enjoy best. I suggest using a Whole Wheat pasta to enjoy added health benefits. You can cook the pasta by placing it in a large pot of boiling water and cooking for eight to ten minutes. Once the pasta is tender, drain and place to the side.

2. Once the pasta is done, you will then want to place a medium sized skillet over a medium to high heat. Add in the olive oil and allow it to sizzle. Once it is warm, add in the onion and cook until it is tender.

3. When the onion is soft, you will want to stir in the tomatoes and the white wine carefully. You will be cooking this for ten minutes or so. Be sure you stir gently, so nothing burns to the bottom of the pan.

4. Finally, add in the shrimp and cook everything together for five minutes or so. The shrimp will turn opaque when it is cooked through.

5. Once the shrimp is cooked, toss it with the pasta, and your meal is ready to be served.

6. For added flavor, try adding your favorite spices and parmesan cheese on top.

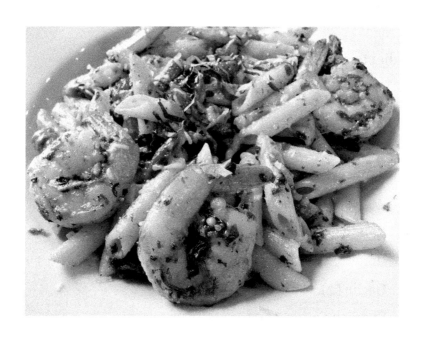

# Mediterranean Flounder

Servings: Four

Time: Forty-five Minutes

Calories Per Serving: 280

Carbohydrates: 8g

Proteins: 25g

Fats: 16g

Ingredients:

- Flounder Fillet (1 Lb.)
- Fresh Basil (6)
- Parmesan Cheese (3 T.)
- Capers (.25 C.)
- White Wine (.25 C.)
- Kalamata Olives (24)
- Italian Seasoning (.25 t.)
- Garlic (2)
- Spanish Onion (.50)
- Extra Virgin Olive Oil (2 T.)
- Plum Tomatoes (5)

Instructions:

1. Before you begin cooking, you will want to preheat your oven to 425 degrees.
2. As the oven warms up, you will want to take a large saucepan and begin to boil water. Once boiling, place

the tomatoes in and then immediately remove into a bowl of ice water. When this step is complete, remove the skins and chop the tomatoes into small pieces. You can set this aside in the bowl when you are done.

3. Next, you will want to heat a medium sized skillet over medium heat. Place the olive oil in the warm skillet and wait until it begins to sizzle. Once this happens, add in the onion and cook for five minutes or until it becomes tender.

4. When the onions are done cooking, you can add in the tomatoes along with the Italian seasoning and garlic. You will cook this mixture for five to seven minutes. At the end, the tomatoes should be nice and tender.

5. Once these vegetables are done, you can mix in the half of your basil leaves, the lemon juice, capers, wine, and the olives. At this point, you will want to reduce the heat and carefully blend in the parmesan cheese. You will cook this for about fifteen minutes. At the end of this time, the mixture should be reduced to a thick sauce.

6. With your sauce completed, you can now place the flounder fillets into a shallow baking dish. Next, pour your sauce over the fillets and top with the rest of the basil leaves.

7. When you are ready, pop the baking dish into the oven for twelve to fifteen minutes. By the end, the fish should flake easily when you press it with a fork.

8. Carefully remove the fish from the oven and serve with your favorite vegetable on the side for a well-rounded and delicious meal.

# Mediterranean Salmon

Servings: Four

Time: Thirty Minutes

Calories Per Serving: 495

Carbohydrates: 10g

Proteins: 37g

Fats: 35g

Ingredients:

- Salmon Fillets (4)
- Salt (.25 t.)
- Pepper (.25 t.)
- Thyme (4 Sprigs)
- Basil Leaves (8)
- Black Olive Tapenade (2 T.)
- Shallot (1)
- Extra Virgin Olive Oil (4 T.)
- Cherry Tomatoes (1 Container)

Instructions:

1. Before you begin cooking, go ahead and preheat your oven to 425 degrees.
2. As the oven heats up, take a small bowl and toss in the cherry tomatoes with the salt, pepper, thyme, basil, shallot, tapenade, and olive oil. Be sure to mix

everything together well so that the tomatoes are evenly coated.

3. Next, you will want to take a baking dish and line it with tin foil. Once this is done, you can place each piece of salmon down. When the salmon is set, cover each piece of the fish with about a fourth of the tomato mixture.

4. When the dish is ready, you will want to fold the edges of the foil over the salmon and seal the edges.

5. Next, pop the dish into the oven and bake for ten to twelve minutes. By the end, the fish should be easy to flake with a fork. The salmon should have a nice pale pink in the center when it is cooked through.

6. Finally, remove the fish from the oven and allow to cool. You can serve this over a bed of rice or with a vegetable for a well-rounded dinner.

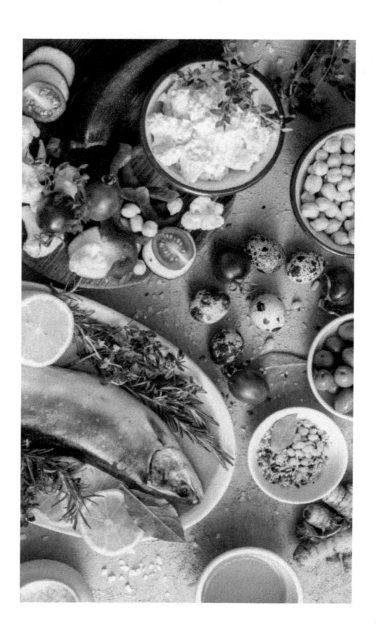

# Chapter Seven: Snacks and

# Desserts Recipes

# Easy Deviled Eggs

Servings: Two

Time: Fifteen Minutes

Calories Per Serving: 330

Carbohydrates: 5g

Proteins: 20g

Fats: 26g

Ingredients:

- Paprika (.25 t.)
- Celery (1 T.)
- Salt (.25 t.)
- Mustard (1 t.)
- White Vinegar (1 t.)
- White Sugar (1 t.)
- Mayonnaise (2 T.)
- Hard-cooked Eggs (6)

Instructions:

1. To begin this recipe, you will want to hard boil your eggs the way you typically do. Once they are done, remove the shell and place on a plate.

2. With the eggs ready, you will want to slice them in half, lengthwise carefully. Once this is done, go ahead and remove the yolks and place them in a small bowl.

3. In the bowl, begin to mash the yolks with a fork. When this step is complete, you can add the salt, chopped celery, onion, mustard, vinegar, sugar, and mayonnaise. Be sure to mix everything together well, so the ingredients are spread out.

4. Next, you will stuff the yolk mixture back into the egg whites. If you want a cleaner process, you can also pipe the mixture back into the eggs.

5. For a final touch, sprinkle some paprika over the top.

6. I suggest refrigerating the eggs until ready to serve or enjoy right away for a delicious snack.

# Apple Chips

Servings: Six

Time: One and a Half Hours

Calories Per Serving: 25

Carbohydrates: 7g

Proteins: .1g

Fats: 0g

Ingredients:

- Ground Cinnamon (.50 t.)
- White Sugar (1.50 t.)
- Golden Delicious Apples (2)

Instructions:

1. To begin, you will want to preheat your oven to 225 degrees.
2. While the oven warms up, you will want to prepare your apple. You can do this by taking the core out and cutting the apple into thin slices.
3. Once this is complete, you will arrange the apple slices on a baking sheet. I suggest putting down tin foil and olive oil to keep the apple slices from sticking.
4. In a small bowl, blend together the cinnamon and white sugar. When this is done, sprinkle the mixture evenly over the apple slices.

5. When you are ready, pop the apples into the oven for about forty-five minutes. By the end, the apples should be dried with their edges curling up.

6. Remove the tray from the oven and allow the chips to cool completely. These are excellent treats for a snack or even a sweet dessert.

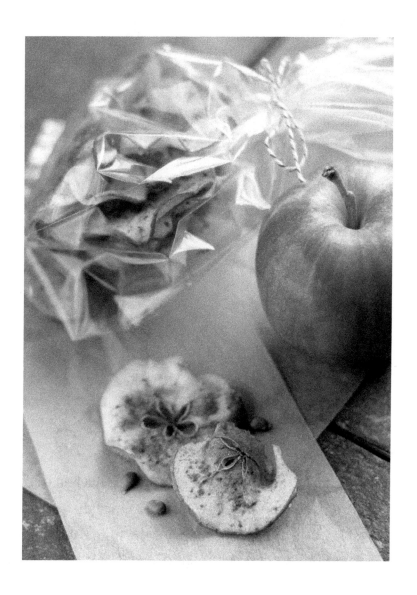

# Stuffed Grape Leaves

Servings: Twelve

Time: Two Hours

Calories Per Serving: 300

Carbohydrates: 30g

Proteins: 4g

Fats: 19g

Ingredients:

- Olive Oil (1 C.)
- Grapes Leaves (60)
- Lemon Juice (.75 C.)
- Chicken Broth (2 Q.)
- Mint Leaves (.50 C.)
- Fresh Dill (.50 C.)
- Onion (1)
- Long-grain White Rice (2 C.)

Instructions:

1. To begin, you will want to take a large saucepan and place it over a medium to high heat. Once the pan begins to warm up, you will place the mint, dill, onion, and rice in and cook for about five minutes. By the end, the onion should be soft and tender.

2. Once the onion is cooked, go ahead and pour in one quart of the broth. When this step is complete, reduce

the heat to low and simmer the mixture for ten to fifteen minutes. At this point in the recipe, the rice should be just about cooked.

3. Now, stir in half of the lemon juice and remove the saucepan from the heat.

4. To create the grape leaf rolls, you will want to take one leaf and place it shiny side down. Once in place, you can insert one tablespoon of the rice mixture toward the end of the leaf. When this is done, be sure to fold both sides of the leaf toward the center and then roll it from the bottom up to the top. You will repeat this with all the eaves, and then you can place them into a four-quart pot. As you place the leaves, try to leave no gaps in-between to help prevent them from opening as they cook.

5. Once all of the leaves are in place, you can pour the rest of the chicken broth over the grape leaves. When this is done, place a cover over the pot and allow the grape leaves to simmer for an hour or so. You will want to assure that the pot does not boil as this will cause the stuffing to burst out of the leaves.

6. Finally, remove the pot from the heat but keep the cover on. Allow these to cool for at least half an hour before serving. Be sure to refrigerate any leftovers; if there are any!

# Goat Cheese and Peach Tartine

Servings: Two

Time: Fifteen Minutes

Calories Per Serving: 480

Carbohydrates: 32g

Proteins: 19g

Fats: 32g

Ingredients:

- Peach Slices (6)
- Salt (.25 t.)
- Pepper (.25 t.)
- Thyme (2 t.)
- Goat Cheese (4 oz.)
- Olive Oil (2 T.)
- French Bread (2)

Instructions:

1. To begin, you will want to turn on the oven's broiler. As this warms up, you can take a baking sheet and line it with aluminum foil.
2. Next, you will want to place your toast on the baking sheet and carefully drizzle a teaspoon of olive oil over the top.
3. When this step is complete, go ahead and take a small bowl to mix together the pepper, thyme, and goat

cheese together. You will want to continue to stir this until the mixture becomes soft.

4. When the goat cheese is spreadable, spread it over each piece of toast until it is completely covered.

5. Finally, place three peach slices on top of the cheese. If desired, go ahead and sprinkle salt and a little bit of olive oil over the top.

6. When you are ready, pop the toast into the oven and cook for about two minutes. By the end, the tops and edges of the bread should be a nice light brown color.

7. At this point, remove the toast from the oven, allow to cool, and enjoy!

# Sweet Strawberry Sorbet

Servings: Four

Time: Two and a Half Hours

Calories Per Serving: 140

Carbohydrates: 36g

Proteins: 1g

Fats: .5g

Ingredients:

- Lemon Juice (3 T.)
- Cold Water (1.50 t.)
- Cornstarch (1.50 t.)
- Salt (.25 t.)
- White Sugar (.50 C.)
- Strawberries (1 Lb.)

Instructions:

1. To start off, you will want to cut the top off of the strawberries and wash them thoroughly. Once you have done this, toss the strawberries into a food processor and blend until they become smooth.

2. Once the strawberries are at your desired texture, take the puree and place it in a large saucepan along with the salt and sugar.

3. Turn the oven on medium heat and cook the mixture from above until it begins to simmer. Once it is

simmering, carefully whisk in the cold water and cornstarch.

4. After a few minutes, you will want to remove the pan from the oven and stir in the lemon juice. Be sure to cool the mixture slightly before placing it in the fridge.

5. You will want to keep this in the fridge for at least two hours before serving.

**Meal Plan**

Below, you will find a meal plan to start with. Please feel free to substitute any meals with the recipes you find most exciting. The meal plan to follow is one to assure you get a few servings of fruits and vegetables in per day. For many people, this can be the biggest struggle. Remember to make this diet your own. The Mediterranean Diet is meant to be enjoyed, becoming healthier should never be a punishment!

As you will soon see, the meal plans to follow include only main meals. If you enjoy snacking through the day, feel free to choose some of the delicious recipes from above. Remember always to drink an adequate amount of water and limit your red wine if you choose to indulge in it. Also, feel free to refer to the grocery list earlier in this book if you have any questions on the foods you can and cannot consume on the Mediterranean Diet.

|  | Monday | Tuesday | Wednesday | Thursday | Friday |
|---|---|---|---|---|---|
| Breakfast | Berry Fruity Yogurt | Healthy Carrot Mini Muffins | Spinach Omelet | Breakfast Zucchini Pie | Banana and Chocolate Vegetarian Smoothie |
| Lunch | Harvest Salad | Cucumber Sandwich | Sweet and Spicy Chicken Salad Sandwich | Lentil Soup | Egg and Shrimp Salad Sandwich |
| Dinner | Greek Chicken with Pasta | Baked Spinach and Feta Pita | Italian White Bean Soup | Baked Zucchini and Potatoes | Mediterranean Stew for Slow Cooker |

|  | Saturday | Sunday |
|---|---|---|
| Breakfast | Black Bean Breakfast Bowl | Veggie Pancakes |
| Lunch | Corn and Black Bean Quesadilla | Greek Quinoa Salad |
| Dinner | Mediterranean Flounder | Shrimp and Penne |

# Conclusion

Congratulations on reaching the end of this book. I sincerely hope that at this point, you feel prepared to begin your diet. It can be daunting, but please feel free to always check back within the chapters of this book for reference. I have tried to provide you with everything you need to get started.

Please remember that the meal plan is just a starting point. As you become more comfortable with the diet, you will be able to extend your knowledge of foods allowed on this diet and can create your own meals. That is the beauty of this diet; it is so flexible! I always encourage testing out new herbs and spices whenever you get a chance!

I hope you have enjoyed this read. I wish you the best of luck on the journey to becoming a healthier version of you. Now go and enjoy the fruits of your labor!

CPSIA information can be obtained
at www.ICGtesting.com
Printed in the USA
LVHW051630010621
689061LV00002B/422

9 781914 916014